Candida Albicans

3rd Edition

Louise Tenney, MH

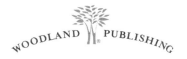

WOODLAND PUBLISHING

For permissions, ordering information, or bulk quantity discounts, contact:
Woodland Publishing, Salt Lake City, Utah
Visit our website: www.woodlandpublishing.com
Toll-free number: (800) 777-BOOK

The information in this book is for educational purposes only and is not recommended as a means of diagnosing or treating an illness. All matters concerning physical and mental health should be supervised by a health practitioner knowledgeable in treating that particular condition. Neither the publisher nor the author directly or indirectly dispenses medical advice, nor do they prescribe any remedies or assume any responsibility for those who choose to treat themselves.

Cataloging-in-Publication data is available from the Library of Congress.

ISBN: 978-1-58054-194-7
Printed in the United States of America

Contents

Candida Albicans: What Is It?   5
An Early Sign of Trouble   6
What Makes *Candida* Grow?   6
    Poor Nutrition   6
    Antibiotics   8
    Hormonal Changes   10
How Does *Candida* Make Us Sick?   10
Types of Candidiasis   11
    Female Yeast Infection   11
    Male Yeast Infection   12
    In the Mouth   12
    In the Gut   13
    Diaper Rash   13
Candida and Pathological System Conditions   14
    The Liver and Kidneys   14
    Allergies   15
    The Immune System   15
Symptoms of Candidiasis   16
Diagnosing Candidiasis   17
Are Drugs the Answer?   18
Natural Therapies   19
    The Importance of Good Nutrition   19
    Other Prevention Considerations   21
    Supplements   21
    Herbal Remedies   24
Summary: Preventing Candidiasis   26
Recipes for a Healthy Diet   27
Appendix: Probiotics and Prebiotics   31
References   32

Candida Albicans: What Is It?

Many people are unaware that they have yeast colonies living in their intestines. Usually, these intestinal yeasts live in harmony with the body through a delicate balance of various types of bacteria. However, a compromised immune system or poor nutrition can upset this balance, allowing the yeast to multiply enough that it takes hold of an area or system. These overgrowths result in a condition called candidiasis.

The most commonly known form of candidiasis is a woman's vaginal yeast infection, an intense burning and itching sensation in the vagina. Because the term "yeast infection" is so frequently associated with vaginal yeast infections, some people don't know that yeast lives in all humans, in any dark and moist environment. Anyone can get a yeast infection in different body systems. The rectum, genital areas, mouth and gastrointestinal tract are areas where yeast typically thrives.

There are approximately 1,500 species of yeast, but *Candida albicans* is the one that most commonly affects humans. Similar to the type of yeast used to make bread, the *Candida* yeast is a small, oval-shaped microorganism that reproduces rapidly by budding. *Candida* cannot thrive by itself, but it flourishes in the intestinal flora of warm-blooded animals.

Candidiasis is becoming increasingly common and widespread. The *Candida* yeast has also become increasingly resistant to conventional medical treatments. But these overgrowths can be prevented if the biochemical balance of the body is maintained. This booklet provides information about the causes of candidiasis, focusing on lifestyle changes that can keep the body in balance and prevent *Candida* overgrowths from occurring.

An Early Sign of Trouble

Candida is just one of billions of microorganisms that live in the body. Its purpose in the body is unclear, although after death, yeast organisms initiate the work of decomposing remains. The small amounts of *Candida* usually present in the intestine do not cause any adverse effects.

When the yeast is allowed to flourish, however, a number of systemic reactions take place, which can make those experiencing a *Candida* overgrowth, or candidiasis, feel downright lousy. Because many of these reactions seem unrelated, individuals may not realize that symptoms like joint pain and heartburn could stem from the same underlying problem. They may even think their symptoms are normal.

Recognizing and treating symptoms of *Candida* overgrowth is vital to the health of the body because candidiasis is an early sign that overall health may be somewhat weakened or the immune system compromised. Healthy immune systems usually keep the yeast from multiplying and causing an infection. When a *Candida* overgrowth occurs, it is clear that something is going on in the body to set the stage for uncontrolled yeast reproduction. Several physiological conditions can make us susceptible to candidiasis. Transplant recipients, people receiving chemotherapy, and those with chronic illnesses are particularly at risk for developing candidiasis due to their already weakened immune systems. For these people, symptoms of candidiasis can also be much more severe.

What Makes *Candida* Grow?

Poor Nutrition

Poor nutrition is the number one contributor to the development of candidiasis, but doctors frequently overlook it when treating these infections. The standard American diet is saturated with more simple carbohydrates (sugars) than the body can process, which has produced a significant increase in serious diseases including obesity, heart disease and type 2 diabetes as well as candidiasis.

The U.S. Department of Agriculture (USDA) estimates that Americans consume an average of 156 pounds of added sugar every year. Added sugars are those that are added to foods or drinks during processing and preparation, not including naturally occurring sugars. A major source of this sugar is sugary treats and the high fructose corn syrup in soft drinks, and processed foods like ketchup and peanut butter and many "low fat" products are often loaded with hidden sugar.

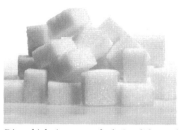

Diets high in sugar feed Candida *and make it easier for the yeast to multiply.*

The human body cannot process this glut of sugar without negative health consequences. One consequence is that the workload of the pancreas is significantly increased, and it sometimes can't keep up with demand. When the pancreas can't process all the sugar consumed, a certain amount of sugar remains in the blood instead of being transferred into cells and used as energy.

Candidiasis is another consequence of sugar consumption. Excess sugar feeds *Candida*, making it easier for the yeast to multiply. Anyone who bakes bread knows what happens to yeast when sugar is added to the mixture. The yeast increases its reproduction, foaming and bubbling at a much faster rate. The same thing happens inside the body when sugar and yeast interact—and this proliferation of yeast leads to infections.

Excess sugar consumption can lead to nutrient deficiencies. In many diets, sugar-laden foods take the place of nutrient rich foods. A lack of virtually any nutrient can predispose the body to candidiasis. Consider supplementing the diet with the following vitamins and minerals, crucial to maintaining a strong immune system:

- Essential fatty acids
- Iron
- Selenium
- Vitamin B_6

- Folic acid
- Magnesium
- Vitamin A
- Zinc

Factors other than nutrition choices can also lead to deficiencies in vital nutrients. These factors include stress, which can deplete the body's store of any vitamin or mineral, and menstruation, which can deplete iron, vitamin B_{12}, calcium and magnesium stores.

The following substances and drugs can also deplete nutrients:
- Aspirin depletes vitamin A, calcium, potassium, B-complex vitamins and vitamin C
- Caffeine depletes vitamin B_1, inositol, biotin, potassium, zinc, calcium and iron
- Chlorine depletes vitamin E
- Fluoride depletes vitamin C
- Nitrate and nitrites deplete vitamins A, C and E
- Sedatives deplete folic acid and vitamin D
- White sugar and white flour deplete B-complex vitamins

In addition, the chemical balance of the body plays a role in susceptibility to disease. An altered acid/alkaline balance can predispose the body to infection. Consuming too much of certain foods can alter the delicate chemical status of the blood. Eating too much acid-forming food, like white flour, cheese and soft drinks, can cause the body to become too acidic. Eating too much alkaline-forming food, like lemons, garlic and onions, can cause an imbalance the other way. Most people are overly acidic, but drastic weight reduction diets that are heavy in just one food group can create an imbalance either way, almost guaranteeing that sickness is just around the corner.

The bottom line is that eating refined sugar and carbohydrates can impair the immune system by inhibiting the body's ability to assimilate nutrients, changing the character of intestinal flora and providing the perfect habitat for yeast to multiply.

Antibiotics

It seems like an oxymoron, but the immune system is actually weakened by the overprescription of antibiotics. Dr. William G. Crook, author of the groundbreaking *The Yeast Connection* (published in 1983 and now expanded into a website, www.yeastconnection.com), and his colleague Dr. Sidney Baker call this a legacy of the antibiotic era of the 1940s and 1950s, when prescription drugs were freely dispensed for almost every sore throat and ear infection.

New antibiotic-resistant strains of bacteria have emerged in

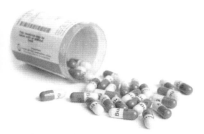

Overgrowths of Candida *frequently follow a course of antibiotics.*

recent years, and many doctors and scientists have concluded that too many antibiotics have been pre-scribed to too many people for too many ailments. While no one would want to be without antibiotics for cer-tain types of infections, their casual and routine use has compromised immune systems and caused the mutation of infectious organisms.

The problem is that antibiotics kill not just bad bacteria, but good bacteria as well. Friendly intestinal flora, which help control the proliferation of bad bacteria, die when exposed to antibiotics. Con-sequently, secondary infections like *Candida* can take over. Using antibiotics for an extended time or taking high doses can make one particularly prone to yeast overgrowths. Broad-spectrum antibiot-ics are especially lethal to friendly intestinal flora. To make matters worse, continually taking antibiotics for something like an ear infec-tion can actually increase an individual's vulnerability to developing another ear infection. This is the vicious cycle of antibiotic therapy.

It is rare to hear a physician acknowledge that the disruption of good intestinal bacteria is one of the side effects of antibiotic therapy, but when friendly flora are killed, there's a price to be paid. Antibi-otics should be used judiciously. If you have a sore throat, ask for a throat culture before you start a course of antibiotics. If the infec-tion is viral, as is often the case, antibiotics are useless against the illness and potentially harmful to the body. Antibiotics are ineffec-tive against viruses, and are often prescribed just because a patient doesn't feel he's being treated if he doesn't get a pill. If more doc-tors cut down on these placebo prescriptions, it will help people's immune systems fight bacteria more effectively.

But even as doctors cut down on antibiotic prescription, giant agribusiness firms are feeding literally tons of antibiotics to cattle and other animals each year so they will fatten faster and bring in greater revenues. Anyone who does not follow a vegan diet can ingest residues of these dangerous chemical additives in meat and dairy products, unless the product is specifically labeled antibiotic- and hormone-free. (See appendix on page 31.)

Hormonal Changes

For women, hormones may play an important role in yeast overgrowth. Prepubescent girls and postmenopausal women are less likely to experience overgrowths. Women taking oral contraceptives and pregnant women, on the other hand, are more susceptible to vaginal yeast infections. This could be due to an increase in the amount of sugar in the vagina, caused by changing hormone levels. Women also seem more prone to

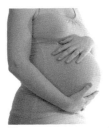

Women are more susceptible to yeast infections when they are pregnant.

vaginal yeast infections at times in their menstrual cycle when progesterone levels are elevated. Apparently yeast reproduces more readily with increased progesterone levels.

How Does *Candida* Make Us Sick?

Candida overgrowth can cause serious disease if it is left untreated and the yeast is allowed to thrive. As *Candida* metabolizes sugar, it creates the chemical byproducts ethanol, acetaldehyde and carbon dioxide. These toxins are released to circulate in the bloodstream, where they cause various problems. For example, they can cause chemical reactions to occur in the body that produce false estrogen. Since this makes the body think it has adequate estrogen, it reduces natural estrogen production. Other toxins produced by *Candida* can deceive the body into thinking it has more than enough of thyroid hormone thyroxine, which can cause menstrual irregularities and hypothyroidism, a condition that affects metabolism.

Ethanol, one of the toxins produced by *Candida*, is an alcohol that is rapidly generated when the yeast has a good source of food, such as high sugar content in the blood. In severe cases, the yeast produces more ethanol that the liver can metabolize. This can cause damage to the liver similar to the effects of drinking too much alcohol.

Acetaldehyde, another byproduct of *Candida*, is related to formaldehyde and causes a variety of malfunctions in the body. It disrupts collagen production, fatty acid oxidation and blocks normal nerve functions.

Other symptoms caused by *Candida* overgrowth are:

- Constipation
- Abdominal upset
- Colitis
- Bad breath
- Mood swings
- Memory loss
- Indigestion
- Depression
- Extreme fatigue

Types of Candidiasis

Female Yeast Infection

Vaginal yeast infections, known in the medical community as vulvovaginal candidiasis, directly affect a woman's quality of life. These infections can cause mood swings, itching and vaginal discharge among other uncomfortable symptoms. Studies show that three in four women will have at least one yeast infection in their lives, and 5 to 8 percent of them will have four or more infections each year.

Vaginal yeast infections can be caused by:

- Chemical douches
- Poor menstrual hygiene
- Spermicides
- Scented toiletries
- Hygiene sprays
- Overuse of tampons
- Alkaline soaps
- Synthetic panties and tights

In recent years, increasing numbers of women have begun experiencing recurrent yeast infections, which worries doctors and scientists. For a small number of these women, each infection has become harder to treat, and medical options are limited. A fairly drug-resistant new strain of *Candida* yeast, *Candida glabrata,* has also emerged. In this modern age when medicine can treat almost anything, *Candida* is getting the better of us. We are headed in the wrong direction. This means that making lifestyle choices to avoid overgrowths of *Candida* are even more important.

Male Yeast Infection

Many men think they can't get genital yeast infections—but they're wrong! It's not just women who experience this uncomfortable problem. Men frequently experience an irritation of the glans penis, an itchy, sometimes painful condition known as balanitis. It usually causes painful redness, swelling or a weeping eruption; it can also cause white patches or blisters. Frequently balanitis causes itching or pain after intercourse. Various things, including trauma, bacteria, viral infections or even overzealous cleaning, can cause balanitis, but it is very commonly associated with *Candida albicans.*

Since yeast flourishes in warm, humid environments, uncircumcised males can experience more of a problem than circumcised (the area beneath the foreskin is an excellent breeding ground for *Candida*), but circumcision does not prevent a yeast overgrowth. Scientists have conducted studies for years examining whether circumcision affects a man's odds for acquiring a penile yeast infection, and have concluded that it doesn't have as much effect as personal hygiene.

A man will not automatically develop a genital yeast infection if he has intercourse with a woman who has a yeast infection. Wash the area after intercourse (whether or not your partner has an infection), but don't be too aggressive, since harsh soaps and detergents can not only irritate the delicate skin but can also lead to yeast overgrowth by stripping away the good bacteria, allowing *Candida* to grow in its place.

In the Mouth

Every dark, humid body cavity naturally has a *Candida* population and the mouth is no exception. A *Candida* overgrowth in the mouth can cause oral thrush. This condition can affect anyone, but it is common in babies (whose immune system takes time to develop fully) and people whose immune system is compromised. Smokers, people who eat a lot of sugar and people with diabetes whose disease isn't well under control also experience a higher incidence of oral thrush.

Thrush starts out localized in the mouth, but can frequently spread down to the pharynx in the back of the mouth or even deeper down the throat into the esophagus. Thrush that has spread in this manner is called oropharyngeal candidiasis.

More than 90 percent of HIV-positive patients experience oral thrush at least once. It is also a common side effect of radiation therapy and chemotherapy since these treatments knock out the immune system, allowing *Candida* to flourish. Thrush can make eating tremendously painful, making an already difficult cancer treatment even worse.

Denture wearers need to be particularly careful because *Candida albicans* can colonize on dental prosthetics. If denture wearers do not carefully maintain oral hygiene, *Candida* can flourish because the plaque that naturally accumulates on the dentures gives it more places to grow. If *Candida* accumulates enough, it can cause a condition known as denture stomatitis, a painful red and sometimes scaly inflammation of the area of the palate covered by the denture. The area can become so inflamed that it bleeds easily. To reduce the risk of denture stomatitis, remove dentures each night and clean them thoroughly. People who sleep with their dentures or don't clean them both thoroughly and regularly have a much higher incidence of *Candida*-related denture stomatitis.

In the Gut

When *Candida* overtakes the other flora in the gut, it can cause a condition called leaky gut syndrome, where the membranes that join the intestinal cells become weak and allow undigested food to leak into the rest of the body cavity. Leaky gut syndrome causes symptoms like bloating, nausea, poor concentration and fatigue. In very severe cases, leaky gut syndrome can lead to larger problems. These include abdominal abscesses (pockets full of fluid, tissue and bacteria) or peritonitis, an inflammation of the membranes that line the stomach cavity causing abdominal pain or tenderness, fever and inability to pass stool. Leaky gut is also the cause of many food allergies as it allows food through that the immune cells recognize as invaders. Even if a *Candida* overgrowth hasn't gotten so bad as to cause a leaky gut, it still negatively affects overall health, causing fatigue, irritability and other symptoms.

Diaper Rash

It can be difficult to tell whether a baby's diaper rash is caused by the usual culprits (acidity in the baby's urine or feces combined with the moist, contained environment and a lack of air) or by yeast. A *Candida*-related diaper rash may look much the same as a diaper rash caused by something else. One prime indication that yeast is to blame is the location of the rash. If it's in skin folds (for example, where the baby's legs meet his pelvis), it's likely yeast-related, because the folds usually keep urine or feces out, protecting against a regular rash. Diaper-area candidiasis can come from the baby's gastrointestinal tract, or exposure from a parent or caregiver. Babies with a case of oral thrush can sometimes also get diaper-area candidiasis.

Facts about *Candida*

- Being irritated by perfume and strong odors is a strong indication of candidiasis.
- Chlorine in drinking water can destroy friendly bacteria in the gut, increasing odds of yeast overgrowth.
- *Candida* can move to different parts of the body and cause immune system depression.
- Since the immune system and the nervous system are connected, *Candida* can invade the nervous system and cause irritability, nervousness, headaches and other nervous system disorders.

Candida and Pathological System Conditions

The Liver and Kidneys

Among their many tasks, the liver and kidneys are responsible for filtering the blood and eliminating toxins—*Candida* among them—through sweat, urine and feces. Diets high in sugar and fats can cause these organs to become so overloaded it is difficult for them to eliminate yeast growth.

A diet rich in vegetables and whole grains can help cleanse the liver, kidneys and bowels and purify the blood, thus helping them filter out excess yeast. Including beans with these vegetables is ideal, as beans are high in protein. Nuts are a great supplement to whole grains, bcause they aid digestion and are high in nutrients and protein.

The following combinations of ingredients can support the liver and kidney in carrying out their detoxifying functions:

For liver cleansing: Combine milk thistle, red clover, dandelion, burdock and parsley.

For bowel cleansing: Combine buckthorn, cascara sagrada, ginger, parsley and black walnut.

For overall cleansing: Make a juice drink combining carrots, celery and parsley, with one clove of garlic and some ginger.

Allergies

When candidiasis causes leaky gut syndrome, the intestines may allow toxins to enter the bloodstream. This may trigger allergies or immune system disorders. A 2010 study published in *Medical Mycology* found that mice with *Candida* colonies had increased incidences of allergic diarrhea.

With children, these allergic reactions can cause learning disorders, behavioral problems and other reactions. The sugar and refined grains found in candy, cookies and white bread can encourage the overgrowth of *Candida*. Even too much fruit juice can lower resistance to *Candida* overgrowths. Children need nourishment from natural foods to develop properly and develop resistance to *Candida*. When they fill up on junk food, they have no appetite for food that will stimulate growth and fight allergies.

A supplement containing the herbs fenugreek, horseradish, mullein, boneset and fennel is helpful for allergies.

The Immune System

Candida weakens the immune system, but it is also more likely to proliferate in an already weak system. The immune system (of which the gut plays a large part) is a unitary bodily system of cells, tissues and organs that defends the body against infection. The immune system recognizes invaders—cancer cells, abnormal or damaged cells and bacteria and viruses that cause infection—and produces antibodies to destroy these invaders. A strong immune system is key to keeping the body healthy.

Besides antibiotics, steroids such as cortisone and prednisone, drugs that suppress acid production, such as H2-blockers and proton-pump inhibitors (used for gastroesophageal reflux disease or GERD) and even birth control pills can weaken the immune system. Other conditions that can significantly damage the immune system include:

- HIV and AIDS
- Liver disease
- Alcohol and drug abuse
- Cancer
- Chemotherapy/radiation
- Diabetes
- Hypothyroidism

Building up the immune system can provide protection from candidiasis. Rest, exercise, eating well and minimizing sugar and yeast are a formula for general healthy living, and a defense against *Candida* overgrowth. The following herbal combinations can help build the immune system:

- A mixture of vitamins A, C and E, selenium, zinc, barley grass juice, wheatgrass juice, asparagus powder, astragalus, broccoli powder, cabbage powder, ganoderma, partheium, schizandra, eleuthero, myrrh gum and pau d'arco
- Combining ginger, capsicum, goldenseal and licorice helps digestion and cleans the lymph system in addition to building the immune system

Symptoms of Candidiasis

Frequently, symptoms of a candidiasis go unrecognized by physicians, resulting in misdiagnosis and ineffective treatment. One woman I interviewed was told by her doctor that she had mental problems and that her condition was psychosomatic. Unfortunately, because *Candida* symptoms are often similarly dismissed or misdiagnosed, many people believe their symptoms are normal, or at least untreatable.

Candida overgrowth can affect various body systems, including:

- Digestive system, causing symptoms such as bloating, cramps, gas, diarrhea, constipation and food allergies
- Endocrine system, causing thyroid gland malfunction (with symptoms like difficulty concentrating, swollen feet and general muscle weakness) and adrenal gland malfunction (leading to feelings of fatigue, constant low blood pressure and persistent allergies)
- Genitourinary system, causing PMS symptoms (mood swings, depression, water retention, cramps, craving for sweets, headaches), vaginal itching and burning, vaginal discharge, recurring vaginal or bladder infections and loss of sexual desire for women and prostatitis, impotence, anal itching and genital rashes for men
- Skin, causing symptoms like eczema, hives, excessive perspiration, acne, psoriasis and nail infections

Diagnosing Candidiasis

Because it can manifest itself through so many seemingly unrelated symptoms, *Candida* can be difficult to spot. A definitive diagnosis involves a positive stool culture or elevated antibody levels. If a physician is uncertain, he or she may take a tissue sample by scraping cells of wherever the discomfort is or culture a tissue sample to determine whether *Candida* is present. Of course, a tissue sample is much more difficult to obtain if the candidiasis is in the gut. Because of the difficulty of diagnosing a *Candida* overgrowth, it often goes undiagnosed. Certain chronic conditions that can accompany an overgrowth of *Candida* include:

- Abdominal pain
- Digestive disturbances
- Muscle aches
- Painful joints
- Headache
- Sense of detachment
- Spots in front of the eyes
- Depression
- Fatigue
- Numbness, burning, tingling
- Mood swings
- Poor memory and concentration
- Sinus congestion

Physicians are now beginning to realize that candidiasis is much more prevalent than previously thought. If you suspect you might suffer from chronic *Candida* overgrowth, you should talk to a healthcare practitioner. However, if he or she recommends drug therapy, consider combining natural alternatives with medical treatment.

Are Drugs the Answer?

Doctors frequently prescribe medications to deal with *Candida* overgrowth, but drug treatment may not be the best way to get rid of *Candida* problems. Since yeast is a fungus, doctors often prescribe antifungals to combat *Candida* growth. The following drugs are commonly prescribed to combat *Candida* overgrowth:

Nystatin (Nilstat or Mycostatin): Nystatin therapy is widely used by doctors for yeast infections. It is available only by prescription in pill, powder and liquid forms. This drug works by damaging the cell walls of the yeast organisms. Although most doctors see it as a harmless drug, it can be toxic to some people and undesirable side effects (diarrhea, nausea, vomiting or stomach pain) are possible. Other possible side effects include a weakened immune system and internal organ damage.

Ketoconazole (Nizoral, Extina, Xolegel, Kuric): This preparation is another widely prescribed antifungal drug, available both in pill and cream forms. The pills can cause liver damage in some instances. Whenever antifungal drugs are used to treat a *Candida* overgrowth, the infection may return when the drugs are stopped.

Butoconazole (Femstat, Gynazole): This antifungal cream disrupts growth of fungal cells, including yeast. It can cause side effects like burning, itching, swelling and increased urination.

Fluconazole (Diflucan): This antifungal antibiotic kills fungi by interfering with their cell membranes. It is used to treat any infection caused by fungus, including *Candida*. Fluconazole is typically taken by mouth. Side effects can include nausea, stomach pain, fever and, infrequently, seizures.

Terconazole (Terazole, Zazole): This is an antifungal cream used to treat vulvovaginitis caused by the *Candida* yeast. Reported side effects include headache, itching, painful menstruation and fever.

Those who rely on drugs to get rid of *Candida* and ignore the root of the problem will likely experience future overgrowths. Concentrating on boosting immunity through a good, nutritious diet that maintains healthy intestinal bacteria is vital, either as a complement to any drug therapy or on its own.

A final note about drug therapy: People who take these medications for extended periods of time sometimes find that their symptoms persist. If this is the case, one should stop taking the drugs and investigate alternative ways to get rid of the infection.

Natural Therapies

The Importance of Good Nutrition

The best approach to candidiasis is prevention. It is far better to keep *Candida* from overgrowing in the first place than it is to treat it. Nutritional changes are the most vital in keeping *Candida* growth under control. An excess of sugar and fat—so typical in the standard American diet—is the worst culprit in fostering the growth

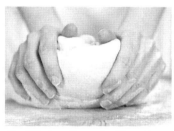

Candidiasis sufferers should avoid consuming foods with yeast.

of *Candida* yeast. Until we acknowledge that what and how we eat profoundly affects how we feel both physically and mentally, all the medicines in the world won't be enough.

While modern medicine has progressed in many medical techniques and experts have found ways to cure life-threatening infections and perform amazing surgical feats, most people have regressed when it comes to the nutritional management of disease. We need to look to our ancestors and incorporate the same types of foods they would have eaten—whole grains, fruits, vegetables and meat only sparingly. These foods will contribute to optimal mental and physical health.

Dietary changes can be difficult, since many people have become accustomed to the ease of preparation and flavor of highly processed, denatured foods that are high in sugar. Eliminating or severely limiting the following foods in the diet can be extremely important in maintaining lifelong good health.

Foods to Avoid

Sugars and foods with high sugar content

- White sugar
- Honey
- Fructose
- Sucrose
- Carbonated soft-drinks
- Dairy products
- Candy
- Maple syrup
- Corn syrup
- High-fructose corn syrup
- Lactose (milk sugar)
- Pretzels and crackers

Fermented, pickled, and yeast- and mold-containing foods

- Alcoholic beverages
- *Saccharomyces cerevisiae* (brewer's/nutritional yeast)
- Cured meats
- Relishes
- Melons
- Yeast breads
- Peanuts and all dry-roasted nuts
- Cider or wine vinegars
- All pickled foods
- Cheese
- Dried fruits
- Green olives
- Soy sauce and tamari
- Mushrooms and all fungi
- Sauerkraut
- Kimchi
- Fermented soy products (miso, tempeh, soy sauce, some soy cheeses, natto)

Fruits

- Citrus fruit (oranges, grapefruit, lemons, limes)
- Pineapples
- Tomatoes

Foods to eat occasionally

- Baked potatoes
- Beans and legumes in small amounts
- Brown rice
- Buckwheat
- Corn
- Millet
- Raw nuts and seeds
- Yams
- Yellow cornmeal

FOODS TO EAT DAILY

- All vegetables except potatoes
- Eggs
- High-fiber foods
- Fish
- Fruits including apples, cherries, pears and all berries
- Kelp, paprika, lemon and cold-pressed oils for seasoning
- Lamb (organically fed)
- Chicken and turkey (organic)

A diet rich in fiber helps the body more efficiently remove potentially harmful toxins, hormones and microorganisms through the intestinal tract and out of the body. The longer these substances remain in a sluggish colon, the more the immune system and other body systems are taxed. Medical practitioners rarely discuss keeping the colon clean, but colon health is vitally important to becoming healthy and resisting disease.

Other Prevention Considerations

For diaper-area candidiasis, the best defense is often a good offense. Change a baby's diaper often and use disposable diapers if possible— they're more air-permeable than cloth and help heal the skin. They are also more absorbent, which is helpful because a moist environment is a good *Candida* breeding ground. Barrier creams can be very helpful in preventing yeast from colonizing on the skin, and occasionally letting the baby go diaperless can also help the skin defend itself against *Candida* colonization. If the rash persists, a topical antifungal cream can be helpful.

Along the same line, women need to be aware that synthetic undergarments trap moisture and bacteria in almost the same way as a diaper. Cotton or organic material is far better for preventing yeast overgrowth.

Supplements

Lactobacillus acidophilus: *L. acidophilus* and other probiotics are crucial for anyone who wants to prevent recurring yeast infections. Acidophilus and other lactic acid producing bacteria help to speed intestinal recovery from antibiotic therapy. Probiotics also help to prevent constipation, which can weaken the immune system. Research has demonstrated that probiotics can slow the growth of yeast organisms. Take a probiotic supplement in capsule or liquid form three times a day.

Amino acids: Amino acids are the organic acids that give structure to muscles, tendons, organs, glands and ligaments. Studies have shown that amino acids interrupt formation of *Candida* cells. Free-form amino acids—amino acids that are unattached to other amino acids—are available in pill form. Free-form amino acids do not have to be digested, so they can be rapidly absorbed into the bloodstream and tissues where they rebuild damaged tissue.

B-complex vitamins: Vitamin malabsorption frequently accompanies infections like *Candida*. Taking a B-complex vitamin supplement can help to offset nutritional depletion and inhibit the growth of *Candida* at the same time. Take the high-potency, yeast-free variety.

Calcium and magnesium: Many people with recurrent yeast overgrowth don't get enough calcium in their diet. Calcium is essential for proper thyroid function. A lack of calcium can also cause headaches, nervous symptoms and fluid retention. Magnesium is necessary to balance calcium. Take 1,000 to 1,500 milligrams of this supplement with vitamin C, kelp and hydrochloric acid for better assimilation.

Caprylic acid: Caprylic acid is a natural fatty acid derived from coconuts. It is an antifungal agent that destroys *Candida* and is considered to be an important supplement for those suffering from overgrowths of *Candida*.

Digestive enzymes: Enzymes help to normalize digestion and break down protein, which can get stuck in the colon. Some digestive enzymes have been shown to kill *Candida* directly and they also work in tandem with antifungals. Some experts especially recommend two particular enzymes: **papain**, a papaya latex extract and **bromelain**, derived from the fruit and stem of the pineapple plant. Use two supplements after meals and two before going to bed.

Evening primrose oil (EPO): This oil contains the essential fatty acid gamma-linolenic acid (GLA) at about nine percent concentration. The body requires GLA for the production of hormone-like compounds that control organ function. Since *Candida* can interfere with the body's ability to manufacture fatty acids, it is a good idea to supplement the diet with fatty acids to offset this effect. EPO can also help prevent *Candida* from becoming systemically invasive.

Garlic: Garlic is an effective antifungal agent and numerous clinical tests indicate that it can inhibit the growth of several different kinds of fungi. It is more potent than several antifungal agents, including Nystatin, in treating *Candida* overgrowth. Garlic can be taken in capsule form. Made from garlic that is freeze-dried to reduce odor, these capsules are taken orally and absorbed systemically.

Garlic in its raw form is pungent, potent and can even burn sensitive skin, but several studies have found that applying a garlic paste to the skin four times a day for 14 days can work as a topical treatment for fungal infections including *Candida* overgrowth. Those who are allergic or sensitive to garlic (or other members of the lily family, such as hyacinths, tulips, onions, leeks or chives) should avoid garlic supplements. Those with a history of asthma, bleeding problems, diabetes, low blood pressure and thyroid disorders should also avoid this supplement. It should not be taken for two weeks before or after any kind of surgery, including dental. *Do not take the capsules if you are pregnant or breastfeeding.*

Olive oil: Cold-pressed oils such as olive oil contain essential fatty acids (GLA, also found in evening primrose oil), which help to balance hormone levels and promote proper sugar metabolism. Essential fatty acids prevent *Candida* from destroying cells. Use at least two teaspoons daily on salads.

Pau d'arco: Pau d'arco is made from the bark of Brazilian *Tabebuia* tree. It has long been used as a folk medicine to treat bacterial infections, cancer, blood coagulation, inflammatory diseases and peptic ulcers. Many herbalists recommend it for a vaginal *Candida* infection because of its antibacterial and antifungal properties. Pau d'arco is also a source of napthoquinones, which promote natural immunity and proper balance in the gastrointestinal tract. Pau d'arco can be taken orally or applied topically.

Psyllium: Psyllium is a grain grown in India that is a popular source of fiber. Psyllium husks provide bulk and lubrication for the bowels and are excellent colon and intestinal cleansers, strengthening colonic tissues and restoring tone. Psyllium can help the body eliminate *Candida* cells after they have been killed by other supplements.

Vitamin C with bioflavonoids: vitamin C, when taken with bio-flavonoids like rutin, hesperidin, Pycnogenol® and grapeseed extract, helps to strengthen body tissues and promote the elimination of toxins. It also helps reduce inflammatory reactions, keeps the immune system strong and controls histamine reactions. Vitamin C can protect the tissues of the body from damage from the toxins released by *Candida*. Be consistent and take a high-quality buffered vitamin C with bioflavonoids daily.

Herbal Remedies

Barberry: The root, bark and berries of this shrub are used for medicinal purposes. Barberry is one of nature's antimicrobial botanicals because its stem, root, bark and fruit contain berberine, an alkaloid that studies have shown to be useful against fungal and bacterial infections. Not only can it treat drug-resistant yeast infections (in conjunction with fluconazole), but it can also prevent the infections from occurring by helping maintain healthy intestinal flora. Healthy intestinal flora also helps to control the diarrhea that sometimes accompanies *Candida* overgrowth. Barberry helps stimulate the immune system by boosting the body's defenses.

Cat's claw: Cat's claw is the common name for several plants, including *Uncaria tomentosa* and *Uncaria guianensis*. Both are used to treat the same symptoms. Found in the rain forest of Peru, this vine derivative can significantly boost the immune system and thus resistance to *Candida*. It is used as a fungicide and has antimicrobial, antioxidant and anti-inflammatory properties. Cat's claw has been used by Peruvians for centuries, and is available in pill, tablet or capsule form. *Patients with kidney problems, heart problems or bleeding disorders should not take cat's claw.*

Dandelion and yellow dock: Both of these herbs grow as weeds throughout North America. Using them together is an excellent way to help the immune system by building the blood's concentration of iron and other minerals. Dandelion flowers, leaves, roots and tops are high in essential minerals and are excellent blood and liver cleansers. Yellow dock root is very rich in easily-assimilated plant iron and can stimulate the elimination of toxins.

Echinacea: This herb, native to North America, is considered a natural infection fighter. *Echinacea* leaves and roots can be particularly effective in treating *Candida* when combined with other herbs and supplements. Augmenting *Echinacea* with garlic, cat's claw, pau d'arco and black walnut creates a potent antifungal elixir.

Geranium oil: Geranium oil is distilled from the above ground leaves of the geranium plant. A 2008 study published *in Biological Pharmaceutical Bulletin* indicated that application of geranium oil suppressed *Candida* growth. Because geranium oil is reputed to affect the endochrine system, *it is not recommended for use during pregnancy.*

When taking herbs and supplements to combat *Candida*, it is not uncommon to experience a sudden surge of symptoms. This is a normal reaction caused by the *Candida* yeast cells dying, referred to as "die-off symptoms." If this happens, you may need to reduce the supplements you are taking to give your body a chance to eliminate the toxins that have accumulated from dead yeast. If die-off symptoms become too bad, take a complete break from antifungals. It can take up to a month for the body to rid itself of so many toxins. Begin taking supplements again when you feel better.

CINNAMON & OREGANO

Two ingredients from typical spice cabinets are also good for fighting *Candida*. Most people think of cinnamon and oregano more as ingredients in delicious meals than as medicine— cinnamon in desserts, fall recipes and drinks, oregano in Italian sauces and other savory foods. But these spices have been used as medicine since ancient days. In a 2008 study conducted on the use of essential oils against candidiasis, published in the *Canadian Journal of Microbiology,* both oregano and cinnamon topped the list of most effective essential oils.

Cinnamon

Cinnamon comes from the bark of a tree found primarily in southeast Asia. It is available as a spice (a dried powder) or as an extract or oil. It's also one of the oldest natural remedies around, having been used in traditional Chinese medicine for years against the flu, parasites and diarrhea.

Although today, cinnamon is used primarily for flavoring food, it also has potent antifungal, antibacterial and antiparasitic properties. It can be used to treat a variety of fungal infections, including *Candida albicans*, and studies have shown that it is extremely effective.

Cinnamon can be made into a tea by dissolving half a teaspoon of cinnamon powder in a cup of boiling water. It can also be taken in supplement form. Ingesting large amounts of table cinnamon is not advised, since this can lead to toxic buildup of certain cinnamon compounds. Extracts in supplements contain the beneficial compounds from cinnamon without the toxic agents in table cinnamon.

Cinnamon oil is much more concentrated than the powder, and in its pure form can cause sores in the mouth or wherever it is applied. While these will heal within days of discontinuing use, it is better to avoid getting them in the first place by not applying it directly to the skin.

Oregano

In the same 2008 study published in the *Canadian Journal of Microbiology*, oregano was found to be the most effective against fungi, including *Candida*. Even yeasts that were resistant to antifungal drug fluconazole were susceptible to oregano.

There are various preparations of medicinal oregano. It is often used in oil form, combined with clove, ginger and wormwood. Oregano's active ingredients are the oils thymol and carvacrol, thought to be potent antifungals. The usual dosage in its oil form is 0.2 to 0.5 milliliters of undiluted oil daily, or one capsule daily in pill form.

Medicinal oregano should not be used during pregnancy due to concerns that larger doses than those normally contained in food may cause miscarriage.

Summary: Preventing Candidiasis

Consumption of sugar is continually rising and conditions like candidiasis will not go away until we eat the foods our bodies really need. Western diets are full of highly-refined grains, sugars and fats, and decades of disastrous eating habits are taking their toll. People who live in more "primitive" cultures and eat a diet rich in fiber, whole grains, vegetables and fruits rarely experience the ailments that afflict more affluent societies. We need to get back to basics and rid our systems of the sweet, sticky foods that not only predispose us to candidiasis but literally "gum up the works" of our bodies and lead to lethal diseases, including obesity, coronary heart disease, diabetes and cancer.

If you suffer, or have suffered, from candidiasis, take action and follow the instructions outlined in this booklet. The results may amaze you. It's hard to cope with life when you feel lousy. When your body receives what it requires to be healthy and strong, your attitude can drastically change.

Remember these tips:

- Keep the immune system healthy with a nutritious diet, regular exercise and supplementation with vitamins, minerals and herbs
- Give up fatty, sugary refined foods
- Avoid cigarettes, alcohol and caffeine
- Don't overuse antibiotics or other drugs
- Take a probiotic supplement every day
- Take a garlic capsule every day

Recipes for a Healthy Diet

Even though dietary changes can be difficult, making these changes is vital to overcoming *Candida* and improving overall health. The following recipes use ingredients that will not feed *Candida* and will help rid the body of this opportunistic yeast.

Bran Muffins

1 cup bran
1 1/2 cups whole wheat or
  pastry flour
1 egg
1/2 cup nut and seed milk (see
recipe on page 28)

1/4 cup tupelo honey
1 cup fresh apples, grated
1 1/4 teaspoons baking powder
2 tablespoons cold-pressed oil
1 teaspoon orange rind

Mix all ingredients together. Spoon batter into greased muffin tins. Bake for 20 minutes at 400°F. Makes 12 muffins.

Seed Cereal

1 tablespoon sesame seeds, ground
1 tablespoon sunflower seeds, ground
1 tablespoon almonds, ground
1 teaspoon chia seeds
1 teaspoon flaxseeds

Soak overnight in filtered water. Cereal will be ready in the morning. Can be eaten with fruit. Makes one serving.

Fish Patties

1 cup tuna fish
1/2 cup cooked millet
1 egg
1 small onion, chopped
1 tablespoon fresh lemon juice
2 tablespoons butter
1/2 cup almonds, ground

Combine tuna, millet, egg, onion, lemon juice and butter. Form into patties and roll in ground almonds. Place on oiled baking sheet. Bake for about 20 minutes at 350°F.

Nut and Seed Milk

1/2 cup almonds
1/2 cup sesame seeds
1/4 cup pecans
1 quart filtered water

Soak all ingredients together overnight in the refrigerator. Blend in blender for three minutes. Strain out the milk and use the remaining grains in grain or vegetable dishes.

Corn Bread

1 1/2 cup cornmeal
1/2 cup whole wheat pastry flour
3 teaspoons baking powder
1 teaspoon sea salt
1 egg
3 tablespoons cold-pressed oil
1 1/2 cups nut and seed milk (see recipe, above)

Combine dry ingredients, beat in egg and add oil and nut milk. Blend together. Bake in a square pan for 25 minutes at 400°F.

Okra Bake

2 cups okra, fresh or frozen
1 tablespoon olive oil
Vegetable seasoning to taste

2 large fresh tomatoes
1 small onion, chopped

Sauté onion and okra in olive oil. Add tomatoes and seasoning and bake in oven for 20 minutes at 350°F.

Raw Vegetable Soup

2 large fresh tomatoes, diced
1/2 cup celery, chopped
1 medium white onion, chopped
1/4 cup parsley, chopped
1 clove garlic, minced
1/2 cup cabbage, shredded

1 quart filtered water
2 tablespoons butter
1 cup carrots, grated
1 cup fresh peas
1 cup pea pods, cut into small
   pieces

Warm the butter in a pan and turn the heat off. Add the tomatoes, celery, onion, parsley and cabbage. Put a lid on the pan. Let it sit. Heat the water to boiling, turn the heat off and add butter and vegetables and season with kelp and vegetable seasoning. Add carrots, peas and pea pods. Warm all ingredients together and serve.

Vegetable Soup

2 tablespoons oil
1 medium onion, chopped
1 clove garlic, minced
1 quart filtered water
2 cups potato skins, chopped
1/2 cup carrots, chopped
1 cup summer squash, chopped

1 cup cooked pinto beans
1 stalk celery, chopped
2 tablespoons vegetable broth
Vegetable seasoning to taste
1/4 cup parsley, chopped
Rye crackers

Sauté oil, onion and garlic until transparent in color. Add water and the remaining ingredients, except parsley and rye crackers, and simmer for about 30 minutes. When cooked, add parsley and serve with rye crackers.

Stuffed Avocados

1/2 avocado for each person
1 red pepper, chopped
1 small red onion, chopped
1/2 cup celery, chopped

1 large tomato, cut in half
Cashew mayonnaise (see recipe, below)
Leaf lettuce

Toss all ingredients with cashew mayonnaise. Serve on a bed of leaf lettuce.

Cashew Mayonnaise

1/2 cup raw cashews
1 cup filtered water
1 teaspoon kelp
1 tablespoon lecithin granules

1/4 teaspoon paprika
4 tablespoons fresh lemon juice
1 cup safflower oil

Blend cashews, pure water, kelp, lecithin and paprika in a blender. Add lemon juice slowly. Pour the oil in a thin stream while the blender is running.

Wild Rice and Vegetables

2/3 cup wild rice
3 cups filtered water
2 tablespoons olive oil
2 stalks celery, chopped
1 onion, chopped
1 green pepper, chopped

2 tablespoons butter
1/2 teaspoon sea salt
1/2 teaspoon kelp
1 tablespoon vegetable seasoning
1 cup chopped almonds

Clean rice. Sauté rice lightly in the olive oil with the onion. Pour rice and onion in the water, bring to a boil and simmer covered for 45 minutes.
Lightly sauté celery and green peppers in butter. Add to rice mixture when done and toss in the chopped almonds.

Appendix: Probiotics and Prebiotics

Probiotics

Probiotics are beneficial bacteria that are found in the digestive tract of healthy individuals. The root words "pro" and "biotics" literally mean "for life." Probiotics can be taken as supplements or consumed in some cultured or fermented foods. When administered in adequate amounts, they can benefit the immune system, the liver, the intestines and even help with bowel regularity. Since probiotics also help control overgrowth of yeast, they are useful in combating *Candida*.

Recently, many companies have been advertising the probiotics found in their foods or beverages. Sales of foods making these claims, like yogurt, have increased dramatically in recent years. Since yogurt is made with live cultures, it is a probiotic food, but this doesn't mean that all yogurt will be helpful in fighting *Candida*. These products typically contain a different strain of probiotic bacteria—usually *Bifidobacterium animalis*.

Kefir, a fermented milk drink, is another source of probiotics, including *L. acidophilus*. While not quite as widely consumed as yogurt, kefir is growing in popularity and can typically be found in the dairy section of the average large supermarket.

There is no standard labeling requirement to help buyers of probiotic products. The word "probiotic" on the label is not enough to tell whether a given product will be effective against candidiasis.

It is important to remember that sugar feeds *Candida*, so look for **unsweetened** varieties that contain *acidophilus*. Capsule form may be the most effective way to supplement the diet with probiotics. It is most beneficial to take *L. acidophilus* supplements on an empty stomach.

Probiotics are commonly used to treat diarrhea, which often follows a course of antibiotics when both good and bad gut flora are wiped out. Studies have shown that probiotics can reduce the duration of diarrhea and reduce the risk of developing inflammatory bowel diseases and intestinal bacterial overgrowth after gut surgery. Studies using probiotics against antibiotic-resistant bacteria (formed when antibiotics are over prescribed, or when people don't take their complete antibiotic course and let the most resistant bacteria live and reproduce) have been especially promising. Probiotics produce lactic acid, which makes the climate of the gut less conducive to pathogenic bacteria.

Probiotics have been found to inhibit the growth of vaginal *Candida albicans* in clinical trials, indicating that an oral dose of probiotics might help prevent recurrent yeast overgrowths. The good bacteria supplied by the probiotics crowds out yeast, returning the digestive tract to a balance that crowds out *Candida*. The evidence available is limited, but this is good news for individuals who have had problems with traditional candidiasis treatment.

An article published in the *American Journal of Gastroenterology* in 2008 cautioned that probiotics could present serious health risks for patients who are immunocompromised. Those with serious health problems should not embark on a probiotics-rich diet without consulting a healthcare practitioner.

Prebiotics

Prebiotics are non-digestible soluble fibers that stimulate the growth of beneficial bacteria in the digestive system by acting as an energy source for these bacteria. They are usually carbohydrates and are reputed to promote the growth of beneficial gut bacteria. Prebiotics are not sugars, which would feed yeast. Rather, prebiotics are a soluble fiber that is not absorbed in the stomach and passes into the bowel where it is fermented by good bacteria—helping prevent an overgrowth of *Candida*. Prebiotics stimulate the growth of good bacteria and increase the body's resistance to invading pathogens.

Wheat, onion, bananas and garlic are sources of prebiotics as they contain fructooligosaccharides (FOS). Raw chicory root and Jerusalem artichoke contain inulins, which are also great sources of probiotics. Other good probiotic sources include soybeans, raw oats and unrefined barley.

References

Buitrón García-Figueroa, R., Araiza-Santibáñez, J. et al. "*Candida glabrata*: an emergent opportunist in vulvovaginitis." *Cirugía y Cirujanos*. 77, no. 6 (Nov.–Dec. 2009): 423–7.

Carrerra, M.A., Donatti, L. "A new model of vaginal infection by *Candida albicans* in rats." *Mycopathologia*. Published electronically June 9, 2010. doi: 10.1007/s11046-010-9326-1.

Chmielewska, A., and Szajewska, H. "Systematic review of randomized controlled trials: Probiotics for functional constipation." *World Journal of Gastroenterology.* 16, no. 1 (Jan. 2010): 69–75

Culligan, E., Hill, C. et al. "Probiotics and gastrointestinal disease: successes, problems and future prospects." *Gut Pathology.* 23, no. 1 (Nov. 2009): 1:19.

Deng, Z., Kiyuna, A. et al. "Oral candidiasis in patients receiving radiation therapy for head and neck cancer." *Otolaryngology—Head and Neck Surgery.* 143, no. 2 (Aug. 2010): 242–7.

Dominguez-Vergara, A.M., Vázquez-Moreno, L. et al. "Role of prebiotic oligosaccharides in prevention of gastrointestinal infections: a review." *Archivos Latinoamericanos de Nutrición.* 59, no. 4 (Dec. 2009): 358–68.

Elkins, R. *Cat's Claw.* Pleasant Grove, Utah: Woodland Publishing, 1995.

Falagas, ME, Betsi, GI. et al. "Probiotics for prevention of recurrent vulvovaginal candidiasis: a review." *Journal of Antimicrobial Chemotherapy.* 58, no. 2 (Aug. 2006): 266–72.

Gibson, G. "Prebiotics as gut microflora management tools." *Journal of Clinical Gastroenterology.* 42 (July 2008): 75–79.

Horowitz BJ. "Sugar chromatography studies in recurrent candida vulvovaginitis." *Journal of Reproductive Medicine.* 29, no. 7 (July 1984): 441–3.

Lee, H.Y., He, X. et al. "Enhancement of antimicrobial and antimutagenic activities of Korean barberry (*Berberis koreana* Palib.) by the combined process of high-pressure extraction with probiotic fermentation." *Journal of the Science of Food and Agriculture.* Published electronically Jul. 29, 2010. doi 10.1002/jsfa.4098.

LeGro, W. ed. *High Speed Healing.* Emmaus, PA: Rodale, 1987.

Lye, H.S., Kuan, C.Y. et al. "The improvement of hypertension by probiotics: effects on cholesterol, diabetes, rennin, and phytoestrogens." *International Journal of Molecular Sciences.* 10, no. 9 (Aug. 2009): 3755–75.

Maruyama N, et al. "Protective activity of geranium oil and its component, geraniol, in combination with vaginal washing against vaginal candidiasis in mice." *Biological Pharmaceutical Bulletin.* 31, no. 8 (Aug. 2008): 1501-6.

Michail, S. "The role of probiotics in allergic disease." *Allergy, Asthma & Clinical Immunology.* 5, no 1 (2009): 5.

Mills, E.J., and Perri, D. et al. "Antifungal treatment for invasive Candida infections: a mixed treatment comparison meta-analysis." *Annals of Clinical Microbiology and Antimicrobials.* 8 (June 2009): 23.

Moshfegh, A., and Friday, J. et al. "Presence of inulin and oligofructose in the diets of Americans." *Journal of Nutrition.* 129 (July 1999): 1407S–1411S.

Murray, M. and Pizzorno, J. *Encyclopedia of Natural Healing.* (Rocklin, California: Prima Publishing, 1991): 186.

Ono, F., and Yasumoto, S. "Genital candidiasis." *Japanese Journal of Critical Medicine.* 67, no. 1 (Jan. 2009): 157–61.

Ouwehand, A., and Nermes, M. et al. "Specific probiotics alleviate allergic rhinitis during the birch pollen season." *World Journal of Gastroenterology.* 15, no. 26 (July 2009): 3261–8.

Pfaller, M.A., and Diekema, D.J. "Epidemiology of invasive candidiasis: a persistent public health problem." *Clinical Microbiology Reviews.* 20, no. 1 (Jan. 2007): 133–63.

Pirotta, M.V., and Garland, S.M. "Genital *Candida* species detected in samples from women in Melbourne, Australia before and after treatment with antibiotics." *Journal of Clinical Microbiology.* 44, no. 9 (Sept. 2006): 3213–7.

Pomarico, L., D., and Ferraz, D. et al. "Associations among the use of highly active antiretroviral therapy, oral candidiasis, oral *Candida* species and salivary immunoglobulin A in HIV-infected children." *Oral Surgery, Oral Medicine, Oral Pathology, Oral Radiology, and Endodontology.* 108, no. 2 (Aug. 2009): 203–10.

Pontes, H.A., and Paiva, H.B. et al. "Oral candidiasis mimicking an oral squamous cell carcinoma: report of a case." *Gerodontology.* Published electronically Jul. 12, 2010. doi 10.1111/j.1741-2358.2010.00371.x.

Pozzatti, P., and Scheid, L.A. et al. "In vitro activity of essential oils extracted from plants used as spices against fluconazole-resistant and fluconazole-susceptible *Candida* spp." *Canadian Journal of Microbiology.* 54, no. 11 (Nov. 2008): 950–6.

Reid, G., and Jass, J. et al. "Potential uses of probiotics in clinical practice." *Clinical Microbiology Reviews.* 16, no. 4 (Oct. 2003): 658–72.

Roberfroid, M. "Prebiotics: the concept revisited." *The American Society for Nutrition Journal of Nutrition.* 137 (March 2007): 830S–837S.

Salerno, C., and Pascale, M. "*Candida*-associated denture stomatitis." *Medicina Oral, Patología Oral, y Cirugía Bucal.* 10, no. 1

(Aug. 2010): 25–31.

Schulze, J. "Yeasts in the gut: from commensals to infectious agents." *Deutsches Ärzeteblatt International.* 106, no. 51–52 (Dec. 2009): 837–42.

Shahid, Z., and Sobel, J.D. "Reduced fluconazole susceptibility of *Candida albicans* isolates in women with recurrent vulvovaginal candidiasis: effects of long-term fluconazole therapy." *Diagnostic Microbiology and Infectious Disease.* 64, no.3 (July 2009): 354–6.

Sharp, R., and Achkar, J.P., et al. "Helping patients make informed choices about probiotics: a need for research." *American Journal of Gastroenterology.* 104, no. 4 (April 2008): 809–13.

Sonoyama K et al. "Gut colonization by Candida albicans aggravates inflammation in the gut and extra-gut tissues in mice." *Medical Mycology.* Published electronically Aug. 31, 2010. doi 0.3109/13693786.2010.511284.

Tasic, S., and Miladinovic-Tasic, N. 2009. "Immunopathogenesis of recurrent genital candidosis in women." *Medicinski Pregled (Novi Sad).* 62, no. 9–10 (Sept.–Oct. 2009): 427–33.

Trowbridge, J.P. and Walker, M. *The Yeast Syndrome.* New York: Bantam, 1986.

White, S.J., and Rosenbach, A. et al. 2007. "Self regulation of *Candida albicans* population size during GI colonization." *PLoS Pathogens.* 3, no. 12 (Dec. 2007): e184.

Wilson Gratz, S., and Mykkanen, H. "Probiotics and gut health: a special focus on liver disease." *World Journal of Gastroenterology.* 16, no. 4 (Jan. 2010): 403–10.

About the Author

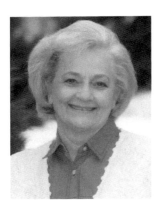

Louise Tenney, MH, has dedicated much of her life to the pursuit of natural approaches to health. Louise has enjoyed immense success as an author, having sold well over a million books. She is also a popular speaker, and has lectured in the United States, Canada, Mexico and even New Zealand. Louise attended Portland State University, where she studied applied chemistry and biology, and earned her master herbalist degree in 1986 from Emerson College of Herbology in Canada. She is the author of more than two dozen books and booklets, including Woodland bestsellers *Today's Herbal Health* (now in its sixth edition) and *The Encyclopedia of Natural Remedies.*